Contents

2 Delegation and Today's RN: Just the Basics
   What is Delegation? 3
   Why Delegate? Today's Nursing Practice Environment 4
   Guidance for Delegation: What You Need to Know Before You Delegate 6
   Education for Delegation 6
   Barriers to Delegation 8

12 Criteria for Delegation Decisions: Six Required Steps
   Assessment of Consumer Care Needs 13
   Development of the Plan of Care 13
   Analysis of Decision to Delegate 15
   Monitoring of Implementation of the Delegated Task 16
   Evaluation of Response to the Delegated Task 17
   Evaluation of the UAP 17

18 Putting It All Together: Decision-making for Delegation by RNs
   Delegation: The RN as a Final Decision-maker 19
   Decision Tree for Delegation by RNs 20
   Discussion Scenarios 21
   Summary: Effective Delegation and You 21

22 Definitions and Terms

24 References

Delegation and Today's RN

Just the Basics

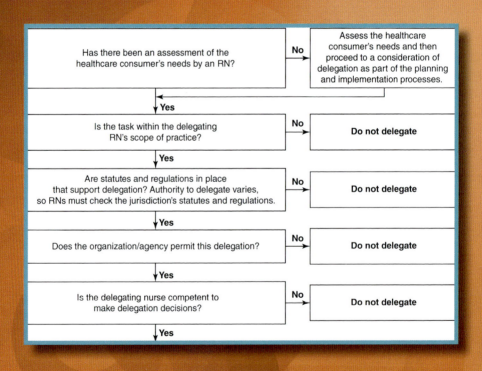

Amy has been a registered nurse (RN) for 5 years, but she is not always sure of what tasks she can, or should, delegate to others. Amy asks Brent, a new PCA (patient care assistant, a type of unlicensed assistive personnel), to draw Mr. Vance's blood for laboratory tests the physician ordered. After two attempts, Brent cannot find a vein that does not collapse. He asks Tim, another unlicensed assistive personnel, to draw the blood. Tim is always able to get the hardest blood draws.

- Did Amy know that it would be difficult to draw Mr. Vance's blood?
- Brent is unable to draw the blood. What should he do?
- Is it appropriate for Brent to ask Tim to draw the blood since Amy initially "delegated" the task to Brent?

What would *you* do in a similar situation? What *have* you done in a similar situation?

The purpose of this booklet is to discuss the process of delegation. Then you will know what Amy, RN, and Brent, PCA, should have known and should have done in this situation. You will also encounter them later in this booklet. The discussion may also further clarify what you should do in a similar situation. *Delegation and You* provides an explanation of principles and relevant strategies for practice in situations in which RNs delegate tasks to unlicensed assistive personnel (UAP).

Delegation also affects licensed practical nurses (LPNs) and licensed vocational nurses (LVNs). Each state's nurse practice act determines which level of licensed nurse is authorized to delegate. (The term *licensed nurse* includes the RN and the LPN/LVN). A licensed nurse may practice to the limit of the scope of practice and licensure. The RN and LPN/LVN must understand the responsibilities and limits of each nursing role in the delegation process (National Council of State Boards of Nursing [NCSBN], 2005). Overarching principles and strategies outlined in this booklet are as defined in the American Nurses Association's (ANA, 2012) *Principles for Delegation by Registered Nurses to Unlicensed Assistive Personnel (UAP)*. ANA recognizes that RNs practice in many settings; therefore, those guiding principles and supporting content are intended to be useful for RNs practicing across the continuum of care.

What is Delegation?

Delegation involves "the transfer of responsibility for the performance of a task from one individual to another while retaining accountability for the outcome" (ANA, 2010a, p. 64). Delegation is a complex process in professional practice requiring sophisticated clinical judgment and final accountability for patients' care. For example, "the RN, in delegating a task to an assistive individual, transfers the responsibility for the performance of the task but retains professional accountability for the overall care" (ANA, 2010a, p. 64). That assistive individual should complete the task or report back to the delegating RN if unable to do so. The task cannot be "sub-contracted" from one assistive individual to another. Only the RN can delegate a task or skill. Unlicensed assistive personnel can assist each other, but the performance of the task or skill must be done by the unlicensed assistive personnel to whom the RN delegated the task or skill.

Nursing judgment, which includes assessment and evaluation, cannot be delegated. For example, when a task or skill has multiple steps that the unlicensed assistive personnel must complete, none of these may include making an assessment or evaluation. The unlicensed caregiver cannot move to the next step or complete the task if assessment or evaluation is involved.

Why Delegate? Today's Nursing Practice Environment

Today's RN faces multiple challenges in providing services to healthcare consumers with complex as well as basic needs. The number of RNs needed continues to increase as the population ages and the healthcare system changes. RNs have worked with licensed and unlicensed staff over the years in providing for the needs of healthcare consumers. The importance of working with others and the abilities to delegate, assign, manage, supervise, and evaluate have never been as critical or challenging, as in 21st century health care.

It is incumbent that the profession of nursing determines when it is appropriate to use delegation in providing care to healthcare consumers. National, state, and regulatory agencies want assurance that delegation is done in a safe and effective manner.

Registered nurses provide culturally sensitive care to consumers. The care provided is safe, timely, efficient, patient-centered, and effective. Nurses provide care in various settings such as acute care, long-term care, community settings, or private homes. Healthcare reform and the advent of accountable care organizations have highlighted the importance of patient-centered care. RNs are essential members of healthcare teams in all settings, along with the consumers, other licensed professionals, paraprofessionals, and assistive caregivers.

> Delegating a task to an assistive individual is a complex part of patient care, requiring the RN's clinical judgment and final accountability. Only the RN can delegate a task or skill.

State nurse practice acts or other statutes define the scope and standards of nursing practice. Individual state nurse practice acts define the legal parameters for nursing practice. Delegation may be addressed in the nursing law, practice act, or statute. The RN delegates or assigns a task based on the physical and mental status of the consumer, considering the potential for harm, stability of the patient, complexity of the task, patient outcome, and the knowledge, skills, and abilities of the personnel to whom the task is delegated.

> **All delegation and assignment decisions are based on the fundamental principles of protection of the health, safety, and welfare of both the patient and the public.**

The RN "is responsible and accountable for individual nursing practice and determines the appropriate delegation of tasks consistent with the nurse's obligation to provide optimum patient care" (Fowler, 2008, p. 156). All decisions related to delegation and assignment are based on the fundamental principles of protection of the health, safety, and welfare of the public. "Such decisions should reflect the nurse's primary commitment to the recipient of nursing and healthcare services—the patient—whether the recipient is an individual, family, group, or community" (Fowler, 2008, p. 150).

Unlicensed assistive personnel and caregivers may perform tasks or activities as members of the healthcare team. LPNs and LVNs may also carry out non-RN tasks. Individual state statutes, policy statements, and professional nursing standards of practice form the framework for clinical practice which includes delegation.

RNs are accountable for the nursing care provided to the healthcare consumer. RNs determine to whom tasks should be delegated, if supervision is needed, and how much supervision is needed. RNs retain accountability for patient outcomes associated with delegation. However, accountability only remains intact as long as the unlicensed assistive personnel carry out the delegated task as instructed.

The modern healthcare environment places more demands than ever on RNs. Patients are more acutely ill, complex, and unstable. Advances in pharmacology and technology place significant demands on RNs. RNs delegate more and more tasks that require increased knowledge and critical thinking skills to delegate effectively. Education and levels of experience of professional nurses present additional challenges to effective delegation. RNs monitor and supervise increasing numbers of unlicensed assistive personnel to determine that safe, quality care is provided. Expectations of unlicensed assistive personnel by the facility or agency need to be consistent. Formal training coupled with consistent expectations leads to a more qualified workforce.

Health care is a dynamic profession. RNs, as members of a collaborative healthcare team, are compelled to be vigilant and action oriented regarding nursing practice and delegation.

Guidance for Delegation: What You Need to Know Before You Delegate

The following provide guidance for the RN regarding delegation:

- The RN is responsible and accountable for the provision of nursing care;
- The RN directs the care provided and determines the utilization of resources;
- The RN may delegate tasks or skills, but does not delegate assessment, evaluation, or the nursing process;
- The RN has knowledge of the organization's policies and procedures regarding delegation;
- The RN considers the knowledge, skills, and abilities of the unlicensed assistive personnel to whom components of care may be delegated;
- The RN utilizes professional judgment in the decision to delegate, taking into consideration the complex care needs of the healthcare consumer, the availability and competence of the unlicensed assistive personnel accepting the delegation, and the type of supervision required;
- The RN acknowledges that delegation involves the concept of mutual respect;
- Nurse leaders are accountable to establish competency requirements related to delegation. Components include assessment, monitoring, verification, and communication;
- The organization is accountable to provide sufficient resources to facilitate delegation which includes an appropriate mixture of staff;
- RNs actively participate in the development of delegation policies; and
- The organization and the individuals involved in the process of delegation share accountability for delegation.

Education for Delegation

Delegation is a skill that should have been part of each RN's basic nursing education, but often is not a specific part of the curriculum. Delegation is a skill that one must learn and practice in order to be proficient. Delegation is not an innate skill but one that develops over time through education, observation, and practice.

Delegation involves critical thinking. Novice RNs are in the early stages of developing the ability to think critically. Delegation is difficult for inexperienced RNs because they have not fully learned how to think like experienced professional nurses.

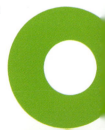

Critical thinking is rooted in what is learned from a basic nursing curriculum. Developed through academic education, many different skills are involved in critical thinking, and improve with experience and repetition. When beginning with critical thinking, most tend to view the world through a personal filter. Over time, a more inquisitive objective view of the world develops as one begins to learn from mistakes, and minor successes form the foundation for larger future successes. A competent RN develops a self-directed consistent process of critically thinking through each care situation. Decisions are based on established standards and result in safe patient care.

> **Organization-based orientation programs should address any specific guidelines and skills that can or cannot be delegated. Scenarios in role-playing setting-specific delegation situations should include critical thinking.**

The process of critically thinking through the steps of the task or skill based on the current assessment of the healthcare consumer, combined with knowledge of the competence of unlicensed assistive personnel, is essential in determining if delegation will be appropriate or not. The decision should always be based on safe patient care outcomes. If in doubt, do not delegate.

Hansten and Jackson (2009) developed a model of self-appraisal of critical thinking skills. The adapted steps include:

- Review the steps you miss when you think;
- Learn from your mistakes as well as mistakes made by others;
- Recognize when your thinking is not optimal. Are you ill? Is the unit short-staffed? Is there a stressful situation at home? All these factors will reduce your ability to focus;
- Present clinical situations to your colleagues for discussion and learning;
- Become a preceptor or mentor;
- Develop an education plan that identifies strengths and areas for growth;
- Trust your instincts. Something may be wrong even though you have no concrete evidence; and

Find and utilize a model for creative thinking and problem-solving. A step-by-step critical thinking process will then become a natural process to you.

Organization-based orientation programs should address delegation and any specific guidelines and skills that can or cannot be delegated. Role-playing delegation situations appropriate to the setting, which include scenarios with critical thinking discussions, are essential to learning. (For more about scenario-based education in delegation, see the section, Addressing Barriers to Delegation, on page 10.)

Nurse managers can set the expectations for appropriate delegation, making sure both the RN and unlicensed assistive personnel are aware of the individual roles. Periodic feedback from the managers is important to assure that appropriate delegation decisions are made. A safe environment/atmosphere is essential for the RN and unlicensed assistive personnel to be able to discuss delegation situations without fear so safe patient care can be maintained.

Barriers to Delegation

Barriers to delegation can be roadblocks to providing appropriate care in a timely manner. Internal and external barriers can exist among all the participants in the process of delegation including the organization, the registered nurse, unlicensed assistive personnel, and the healthcare consumer.

Organization

Organization-related barriers to delegation may include:

- The organization may not have the appropriate staffing mix to allow appropriate delegation to occur. This could mean that the unlicensed assistive personnel are assigned to too many RNs and healthcare consumers to be effective in completing anything beyond the basic care duties of the assignment;
- The organization may not have established guidelines for appropriate skills that can be delegated; and
- The knowledge, skills, and ability of the unlicensed assistive personnel may not have been taught or documented through orientation or training for delegable skills.

Registered Nurses

> Basic UAP skills and guidelines for delegable skills, as well as documentation of UAP competency, should be established and reviewed periodically for appropriateness or any needed additions or deletions.

RNs may be reluctant to delegate because of internal or external barriers. These include when the RN:

- Fears making mistakes (for instance: the RN is new in the RN role or new to delegating);
- Has never worked with unlicensed assistive personnel and does not know how to develop them or work with them as team members;
- Is reluctant to let go of certain aspects of RN work and has a lack of trust in unlicensed assistive personnel or feels a loss of control;
- Is unsure of the skills of the unlicensed assistive personnel and is fearful of errors;
- Does not want to take the time to explain, observe, and evaluate the unlicensed assistive personnel and feels she or he can do it quicker;
- Is inexperienced in using authority to delegate and set expectations for accountability and responsibility with unlicensed assistive personnel;
- Fears being disliked by unlicensed assistive personnel for delegating skills, which may set the stage for lateral violence; and
- Fears that healthcare consumers will think the RN, not the unlicensed assistive personnel, should be taking care of them.

Unlicensed Assistive Personnel

The unlicensed assistive personnel may have no past experience or bad experiences in delegation. Other unlicensed assistive personnel barriers could be that a given member of the UAP staff:

- Is new to role as unlicensed assistive personnel and lacks confidence;
- Lacks skills competency;
- Is disorganized;
- Is dependent on constant direction;
- Avoids responsibility beyond the basics;
- Is overloaded by work, or is assigned to work with multiple RNs and healthcare consumers with too many delegated tasks/skills to accomplish;
- Fears making mistakes;
- Has conflicts with the RN, which again may set the stage for lateral violence. The RN may expect more from the unlicensed assistive personnel than the person is able to give. The background and experience of the unlicensed assistive personnel may be insufficient to carry out the assigned task/skill. The RN may not give the unlicensed person the opportunity to learn; and
- Doesn't want to be held accountable.

Healthcare Consumers

Healthcare consumers and their family members may be fearful of mistakes occurring if an RN doesn't perform the skill. They may be unaware that unlicensed assistive personnel are competent and permitted to perform certain skills.

Addressing Barriers to Delegation

Scenario-based education with joint discussion between RNs and unlicensed assistive personnel provides an opportunity for increased understanding of the roles and responsibilities in delegation. Open discussion regarding the barriers to delegation could result in removing most of the barriers.

The organization's nursing leadership needs to endorse and support delegation in order for it to be used in the practice setting. Basic unlicensed assistive personnel skills and guidelines for delegable skills should be established and reviewed periodically to determine appropriateness or need for additions or deletions. Documentation of unlicensed assistive personnel competency should occur at least annually and as needed.

Opportunities for development of the RN and unlicensed assistive personnel in using the process of delegation should occur during orientation to the organization and with continuing education throughout their employment. Emphasis on the authority of the RN to delegate along with the accountability and responsibility for both the RN and unlicensed assistive personnel are important to successful delegation. The education should clearly outline the policies, procedures, and protocols specific to delegation. Customized scenarios are often effective in showing examples of correct and incorrect delegation. The scenarios can be starting points in offering opportunities for discussion with questions and answers facilitated by a knowledgeable RN educator or staff preceptor.

> The LPN/LVN on the team may assign or delegate nursing tasks/skills to the UAP, and must consider the same criteria as the RN before delegating any task/skill to the UAP.

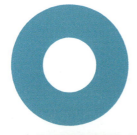

Delegation: The RN and the LPN/LVN

The RN may delegate to the LPN/LVN as well as to unlicensed assistive personnel. The RN and the LPN/LVN need to be aware of their specific state's scope of practice for the LPN/LVN. The LPN/LVN practices under the direction of a licensed professional nurse, licensed physician, or licensed dentist (as examples) and does not require the specialized knowledge, skills, abilities, or judgment required in professional nursing. An LPN/LVN may assign nursing activities within the LPN/LVN scope of practice to other LPNs/LVNs and may delegate nursing tasks/skills to unlicensed assistive personnel. The LPN/LVN cannot assign or delegate care to the RN. In maintaining accountability for the delegation, the LPN/LVN must consider the same criteria as the RN before delegating any task/skill to the UAP.

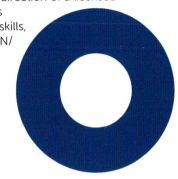

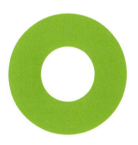

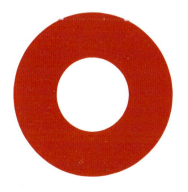

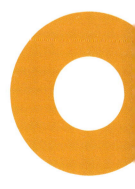

Criteria for Delegation Decisions
Six Required Steps

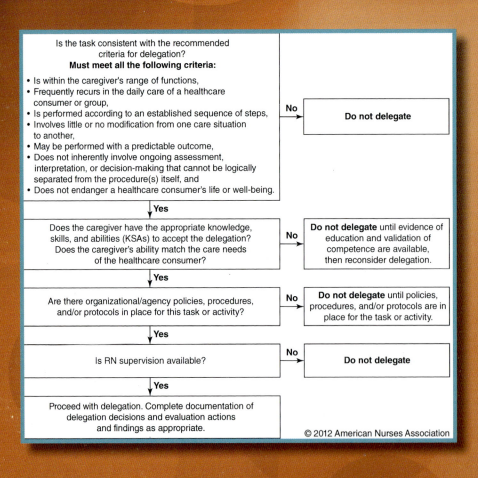

To determine if delegation is appropriate, the RN must perform this six-step process (ANA, 2012, pg. 9–10):

1. Perform an assessment of the healthcare consumer's care needs;
2. Develop a plan of care with the healthcare consumer and family;
3. Perform an analysis;
4. Monitor implementation of the delegated task as appropriate to the overall plan of care;
5. Evaluate the overall condition of the healthcare consumer and the consumer's response to the delegated task; and
6. Evaluate the unlicensed assistive personnel's skills and performance of tasks and provide feedback for improvement if needed.

Assessment of Consumer Care Needs

1. Perform an assessment of the healthcare consumer's care needs.

- Determine if any cultural modifications are required. Talk to the healthcare consumer and family members to identify any modifications that are necessary to meet their cultural needs. Document the necessary modifications and inform the unlicensed assistive personnel of how to incorporate the modifications to meet the healthcare consumer's needs.
- Determine if the healthcare consumer's condition is stable and predictable. If the healthcare consumer's condition is unstable, the unlicensed assistive personnel may not be able to follow exacting steps in performing the delegable skill. The RN may need to make judgments based on an ongoing assessment of the healthcare consumer and alter the plan of care.
- Assess the environment where care will be provided. If the environment in which care will be provided is stable, the unlicensed assistive personnel should perform the delegable skill. If the skill required needs to be performed under unstable emergent conditions alterations may be required and should be done by the RN.

Development of the Plan of Care

2. Develop a plan of care with the healthcare consumer and family.

- Identify the tasks that can be delegated.
  - ❒ Each organization should have a list of basic tasks and delegable skills that can be performed by competent unlicensed assistive personnel. If the skill is outside the RN scope of practice, or prohibited by the organization, it cannot be delegated to unlicensed assistive personnel.

- ❏ According to the NCSBN Five Rights of Delegation (1997), generally, appropriate activities for consideration in delegation decision-making include those:

  - ➤ That frequently reoccur in the daily care of a client or group of clients;
  - ➤ That do not require the unlicensed assistive personnel to exercise nursing judgment;
  - ➤ That do not require complex and/or multi-dimensional application of the nursing process;
  - ➤ For which the results are predictable and the potential risk is minimal; and
  - ➤ That utilize a standard and unchanging procedure.

- Involve and educate healthcare consumers and families about appropriate expectations of the roles of unlicensed assistive personnel and how the expectations will promote a safe environment and improve patient outcomes.

  The RN coordinates the care for the healthcare consumer and is responsible for communicating how the nursing care will be carried out, and by whom on the nursing team. It is important that healthcare consumers know who their care providers are and that the healthcare consumers are treated with dignity and respect.

- The plan of care should include a baseline status of the healthcare consumer.

  The RN has the responsibility for assessment, planning, evaluation, and making nursing judgments on the healthcare consumer's baseline.

- Steps of the task that cannot be changed should be outlined.

  The unlicensed assistive personnel should follow a step-by-step procedural outline for delegable skills established by the organization.

- The unlicensed assistive personnel needs to know who to report to if the baseline status changes.

  The RN must communicate directions to the unlicensed assistive personnel including any special patient needs as well as clear expectations regarding what to do, what to report, and when to ask for assistance. Changes in the healthcare consumer's status require judgment; the unlicensed assistive personnel should notify the RN whenever they note a change in the healthcare consumer's status.

- Document expectations.

  Following organizational documentation policies, the RN may document expectations for performance of the unlicensed assistive personnel in the delegated skills. This may be part of the skills validation process. The RN needs to set expectations for communication from the unlicensed assistive personnel regarding the outcomes of the delegated skills throughout the assigned work period. The unlicensed assistive personnel are responsible for documentation of the skills performed and the healthcare consumer's response.

Analysis of Decision to Delegate

3. Perform an analysis of key factors for the decision to delegate.

- **Is the task or skill within the delegating RN's scope of practice?**

    The RN cannot delegate a task or skill that is not within the nursing scope of practice. Components of care may be delegated, but the nursing process itself may not be delegated. The functions of assessment, planning, evaluation and nursing judgment cannot be delegated. The RN must also follow any organizational guidelines for delegable tasks/skills to unlicensed assistive personnel.

- **Are there federal or state laws, rules, or regulations that support the delegation?**

    The RN needs to be knowledgeable of the state nurse practice act in the state where the RN practices because states may differ in the rules of delegation. The RN has the responsibility to practice nursing within the law. Delivery of care is increasingly crossing state lines, therefore, the RN may deliver care to a consumer in a neighboring state (i.e., telemedicine, call centers). The RN still maintains the responsibility to be knowledgeable of the laws, statutes, and regulations of both the RN's and the consumer's states and to practice within those parameters.

- **Does the employing organization/agency of the delegating RN and unlicensed assistive personnel permit the delegation?**

    Organizations should empower RNs to use delegation as part of their role to meet the multiple needs of their healthcare consumers. Nursing leadership and staff nurses must work together to ensure that the process of delegation is appropriate and complete. The safety and protection of the healthcare consumer should ultimately prevail when using delegation and delivering nursing care. Each organization or agency should define expectations for delegation. Nursing governance councils are a place to start if no current policy regarding delegation exists. Procedures should be developed so that both licensed and unlicensed nursing personnel understand their roles regarding delegation.

- **Is the delegating RN competent to make the delegation decision?**

    The RN must be licensed in the state where nursing is being practiced. The nurse needs to be employed by the organization and have completed the steps above to be competent to make delegation decisions regarding the unlicensed assistive personnel performing a skill for the healthcare consumer.

- **Is the unlicensed assistive personnel competent to perform the delegated task?**

    The unlicensed assistive personnel should have successfully completed the organization orientation which validated knowledge, skills and ability to perform a defined list of basic skills. Specific patient care areas may have added additional skills that are determined to be appropriate for unlicensed assistive personnel. There should be documentation available to the RN regarding the competency of the unlicensed assistive personnel especially if the RN is not familiar with the competence of the unlicensed assistive personnel. The RN assessments of the environment, the healthcare consumer, and the knowledge of the unlicensed assistive personnel are crucial to make sure the delegation is appropriate.

- **Is RN supervision of the unlicensed assistive personnel available?**

  ❏ The delegating RN is responsible for determining the level of supervision needed for the specific situation, and for implementing that supervision, which includes how to follow-up if there is a problem or if the situation changes, requiring the RN to assess and make a judgment.

  ❏ Supervision based on the environment may be on-site or off-site. On-site supervision is when the supervising RN is physically present and immediately available to the unlicensed assistive personnel.

  > **Example:** The delegating RN, Amy, is providing care to Mr. Glover while Brent, PCA, (unlicensed assistive personnel) is providing care to Mr. Fields in another room. Brent can stop what he is doing to get Amy to come assess Mr. Fields if needed. Otherwise Brent will perform the skill, document the performance of the skill, observations, and patient response, and report to Amy.

  ❏ Off-site supervision is the availability of the supervising RN through various means of communication such as written, verbal, electronic, or through telemedicine.

  > **Example:** The delegating RN, Janet, is a school nurse located at the high school who has delegated to Shelly, a school aide (unlicensed assistive personnel), at the elementary school, to administer an inhaler to the healthcare consumer. Shelly has performed this skill competently before and will communicate with Janet by phone if needed. Otherwise, Shelly will document that the skill was performed and how the healthcare consumer responded.

Monitoring of Implementation of the Delegated Task

4. Monitor implementation of the delegated task as appropriate to the overall plan of care.

The delegating RN is responsible for setting the expectations regarding monitoring. Monitoring, or supervision, can be done through observation or communication (i.e., verbal, written, electronic, or telemedicine). It can be a mixture of communication with the unlicensed assistive personnel throughout the given work period they are assigned together. Both parties should be open and receptive to the chosen communication form.

Evaluation of Response to the Delegated Task

5. Evaluate the overall condition of the healthcare consumer and the consumer's response to the delegated task.

Based on the environment, the delegating RN may have the opportunity to visualize and evaluate the healthcare consumer's response to the delegated task, or may rely on documentation done by the unlicensed assistive personnel. Feedback from the healthcare consumer is always important to the evaluation of care provided, and may be immediate or given later.

> **Example:** When Amy, RN, gave Mr. Vance his medication, she looked at his venipuncture sites from the earlier blood draw attempts and saw that they were no longer reddened or swollen. Mr. Vance said the ice pack was helpful and that his arm felt fine now.
>
> **Example:** Janet, School RN, read the unlicensed assistive personnel documentation that charted the administration of the inhaler to the elementary student and that the student said she could breathe better. Later, at a school conference, the student's mother stated how she appreciated that the school could make sure her daughter got the inhaler when needed at school.

Evaluation of the UAP

6. Evaluate the unlicensed assistive personnel's skills and performance of tasks and provide feedback for improvement if needed.

Once the unlicensed assistive personnel has successfully completed an organizational orientation and the knowledge, skills, and abilities to perform tasks and skills for the role have been documented, evaluation still continues. The RN working with unlicensed assistive personnel is in the position to evaluate and document performance of any assigned tasks or delegated skills. Some organizations require annual documentation of designated skills. Feedback for skills performance should be done with mutual respect and upholding the dignity of both parties. Constructive feedback for unsatisfactory performance of a skill should always be given in private behind closed doors with appropriate documentation. A written plan for remediation should be developed by the manager.

Putting It All Together

Decision-making for Delegation by RNs

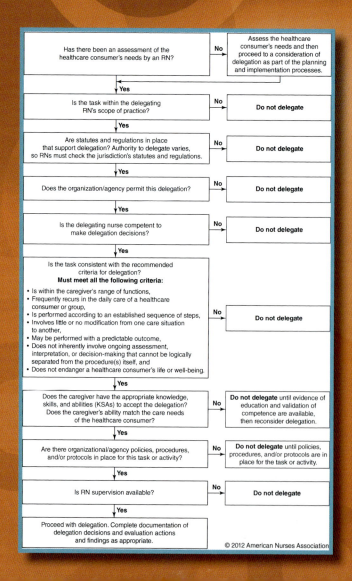

Delegation: The RN as a Final Decision-maker

The nursing profession has several valuable foundational documents that address the role of the RN and delegation. Examples include: *ANA's Principles for Delegation* (ANA, 2012), *Code of Ethics for Nurses with Interpretive Statements* (ANA, 2001), *Nursing: Scope and Standards of Practice, 2nd Edition* (ANA, 2010a), and *Nursing's Social Policy Statement: The Essence of the Profession* (ANA, 2010b). A decision tree for RN delegation was developed as part of *Principles for Delegation,* and is included on the next page to assist you in your delegation work.

The nurse must not engage in practices prohibited by law or delegate to others if prohibited by law. This is consistent with *Code of Ethics for Nurses with Interpretive Statements* (ANA, 2001). The nurse is expected to be knowledgeable about:

- the principles of delegation,
- the risks, benefits, and specific state laws, and
- the regulations governing nursing practice.

This booklet is designed to explore and clarify the process of delegation and to provide overarching principles and relevant strategies for practice in situations in which RNs delegate tasks to unlicensed assistive personnel. RNs must check with their state board of nursing to ascertain state-specific differences related to delegation. The final professional decision to proceed with delegation to unlicensed assistive personnel ultimately rests with the RN.

Let's return to Amy, RN, Brent, PCA, and Tim, PCA. Now that you know the definition and implications of delegation, what should have occurred?

- Amy should have taken into consideration the fact that Brent was a new PCA before she asked him to draw the blood. She should have asked a more experienced PCA, perhaps Tim, to draw the blood since she knew Mr. Vance had fragile veins.
- Brent should not have asked Tim to draw the blood. The "delegation" was not within Brent's practice area. Brent should have gone back to Amy to let her know he could not get the blood drawn and suggest that Tim could draw the blood.
- Tim should not have drawn the blood for Brent. Tim should have asked Amy if he should proceed with the task.

Decision Tree for Delegation by RNs

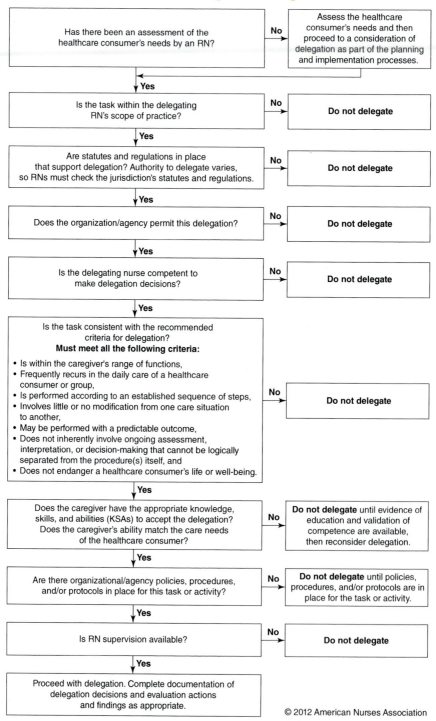

© 2012 American Nurses Association

Discussion Scenarios

Are you able to discuss how and why the other decisions should have been made? Are you better prepared to delegate now that you've read this booklet, including the decision tree? Let's see...

Scenario 1: A middle school student needs insulin before lunch. How will the decision tree help the school nurse decide whether or not to have the teacher's assistant administer the insulin to the student?

Is the non-nurse legally able to administer the medication to a student? The RN must be knowledgeable of state regulations. If the state permits the administration of the medication, is the assistant competent to perform the task?

Scenario 2: A new RN is the nurse manager of a unit at an extended care nursing facility. An LPN with 20 years of experience tells the RN not to worry; she'll take care of everything. The LPN states she will assess all the residents and document the findings, do all the dressing changes, and give all of the medications. What should the RN do?

Scenario 3: A patient has a clean, non-sterile dressing that needs to be changed. How will the decision tree help the RN decide whether or not to delegate the dressing change to the unlicensed assistive personnel?

The RN must first assess the patient and the level of difficulty of the dressing change. Is the task within the practice area of unlicensed assistive personnel? Is delegation permitted in the organization? Is the delegating RN competent to delegate? Finally, is the unlicensed assistive personnel competent to perform the task?

Summary: Effective Delegation and You

The dynamics of a continuously changing healthcare climate and the expectations of the nursing profession compel RNs, as members of the interprofessional healthcare team, to be vigilant and action-oriented regarding nursing practice and RN delegation. Effective delegation requires knowledge and skills to match the task to be carried out with the person to whom the task will be delegated. RNs must be knowledgeable about the principles for delegation, any associated risks and benefits, and specific state laws and regulations governing practice. RNs determine if the unlicensed members of the healthcare team have the appropriate knowledge, skills, and abilities to perform the delegated task. RNs retain accountability for patient outcomes associated with nurse delegation, provided the person to whom the task was delegated performed the task as instructed. Challenges in today's healthcare environment place greater demands on RNs to have the knowledge and critical thinking skills to effectively delegate to others.

Definitions and Terms

The definitions and terms have been taken directly from, to maintain consistency.

Accountability. "Accountability is both related to answerability and responsibility. Accountability is judgment and action on the part of the nurse for which the nurse is answerable to self and others for those judgments and actions. Responsibility refers to the specific accountability of liability associated with the performance of duties of a particular nursing role and may, at times, be shared in the sense that a portion of responsibility may be seen as belonging to another who was involved in the situation" (Fowler, 2008. p. 44).

Assessment. "A systematic, dynamic process by which the registered nurse, through interaction with the patient, family, groups, communities, populations, and healthcare providers, collects and analyzes data" (ANA, 2010a, p. 63).

Assignment. The distribution of work that each staff member is responsible for during a given work period.

Authority. "Authority is the right to act in areas where one is given and accepts responsibility" (Miller & Wright, 2007, p. 34). RNs have authority, or legitimate power, to analyze assessments, plan nursing care, evaluate nursing care, and exercise nursing judgment.

Caregiver. A family member, significant other, neighbor, friend, or other unlicensed designated individual who assists in the care, activities of daily living, or other healthcare activities of individuals with physical disabilities or mental impairments.

Critical thinking. "Critical thinking in nursing is an essential component of professional accountability and quality nursing care. Critical thinkers in nursing exhibit these habits of the mind: confidence, contextual perspective, creativity, flexibility, inquisitiveness, intellectual integrity, intuition, open-mindedness, perseverance, and reflection. Critical thinkers in nursing practice the cognitive skills of analyzing, applying standards, discriminating, information seeking, logical reasoning, predicting and transforming knowledge" (Scheffer & Rubenfeld, 2000, p. 357).

Delegation. Delegation generally involves assignment of the performance of activities or tasks related to patient care to unlicensed assistive personnel while retaining accountability for the outcome. The registered nurse cannot delegate responsibilities related to making nursing judgments. Examples of nursing activities that cannot be delegated to unlicensed assistive personnel include assessment and evaluation of the impact of interventions on care provided to the patient (adapted from Fowler, 2008, p. 49). Delegation involves "the transfer of responsibility for the performance of a task from one individual to another while retaining accountability for the outcome. Example: the RN, in delegating a task to an assistive individual, transfers the responsibility for the performance of the task but retains professional accountability for the overall care" (ANA, 2010a, p. 64).

Healthcare consumer. "The person, client, family, group, community, or population who is the focus of attention and to whom the registered nurse is providing services as sanctioned by the state regulatory bodies" (ANA, 2010a, p. 65).

Nursing process. "A critical thinking model comprising the integration of singular, concurrent actions of these six components: assessment, diagnosis, identification of outcomes, planning, implementation, and evaluation" (ANA, 2010b, p. 41).

Responsibility. Responsibility involves liability with the performance of duties in a specific role (ANA, 2001). Responsibility is a two-way process that is both allocated and accepted (adapted from Miller & Wright, 2007, p. 34; Weydt, 2010). Assistive personnel accept responsibility when they agree to perform an activity delegated to them (Weydt, 2010).

Supervision. Supervision is the active process of directing, guiding, and influencing the outcome of an individual's performance of a task. Similarly, NCSBN defines supervision as the provision of guidance or direction, oversight, evaluation, and follow-up by the licensed nurse for the accomplishment of a delegated nursing task by assistive personnel. Individuals engaging in supervision of patient care should not be construed to be managerial supervisors on behalf of the employer under federal labor law (ANA & NCSBN, 2006).

Unlicensed assistive personnel (UAP). An umbrella term to describe a job class of paraprofessionals who assists individuals with physical disabilities, mental impairments, and other healthcare needs with their activities of daily living and provide care—including basic nursing procedures—all under the supervision of a registered nurse, licensed practical nurse, or other healthcare professionals. UAP may include institutional titles such as, patient care assistant (PCA), certified nursing assistant (CNA), nursing assistant (NA), patient care technician (PCT), school aide, health aide, or care companion. They provide care for healthcare consumers in need of their services in hospitals, long-term care facilities, outpatient clinics, schools, private homes, and other settings. Unlicensed assistive personnel by definition do not hold a license or other mandatory professional requirements for practice, though many hold various certifications.

References

American Nurses Association. (2001). *Code of ethics for nurses with interpretive statements*. Washington, DC: American Nurses Publishing.

American Nurses Association. (2010a). *Nursing: Scope and standards of practice* (2nd ed.). Washington, DC: American Nurses Publishing.

American Nurses Association. (2010b). *Nursing's social policy statement: The essence of the profession*. Washington, DC: American Nurses Publishing.

American Nurses Association. (2012). *Principles for delegation by registered nurses to unlicensed assistive personnel*. Washington, DC: American Nurses Publishing.

American Nurses Association & National Council of State Boards of Nursing. (2006). *Joint statement on delegation*. Retrieved from https://www.ncsbn.org/Joint_statement.pdf

Fowler, M. D. (Ed.). (2008). *Guide to the code of ethics for nurses: Interpretation and application*. Washington, DC: American Nurses Publishing.

Hansten, R., & Jackson, M. (2009). *Clinical delegation skills: A handbook for professional practice* (4th ed.). Burlington, MA: Jones & Bartlett Learning.

Heaslip, P. (1993). *Critical thinking and nursing*. Retrieved from http://www.criticalthinking.org/pages/critical-thinking-and-nursing/834

Miller, D., & Wright, D. (Eds.). (2007). *Leading an empowered organization manual*. Minneapolis, MN: Creative Healthcare Management.

National Council of State Boards of Nursing. (1997). *The five rights of delegation*. Retrieved from https://www.ncsbn.org/fiverights.pdf

National Council of State Boards of Nursing. (2005). *Working with others: A position paper*. Retrieved from https://www.ncsbn.org/Working_with_Others.pdf

Scheffer, B. K., & Rubenfeld, M. G. (2000). A consensus statement on critical thinking in nursing. *Journal of Nursing Education, 39*, 352–359.

Weydt, A. (2010, May 31). Developing delegation skills. *Online Journal of Issues in Nursing, 15*. doi: 10.3912/OJIN.Vol15No02Man01